I BEAT BREAST CANCER FOREVER

How To Conquer Breast Cancer For Life

Gladwell Asher

TABLE OF CONTENTS

INTRODUCTION

Breast cancer originates from abnormal growth of cells in the breast tissue. It is the predominant cancer among women worldwide, although it can also affect men. This condition arises when abnormal cells in the breast start multiplying uncontrollably, resulting in the formation of a tumor. There are two types of tumors: malignant tumors, which are cancerous, and benign tumors, which are non-cancerous.

There are various types of breast cancer, with the most prevalent being ductal carcinoma, which originates in the cells lining the milk ducts, and lobular carcinoma, which begins in the lobules responsible for milk production. Less common types include inflammatory breast cancer and triple-negative breast cancer.

Several factors contribute to the risk of developing breast cancer, including age, family history, genetic mutations (such as BRCA1 and BRCA2), hormonal influences, lifestyle choices (such as alcohol consumption and obesity), and exposure to specific environmental factors.

Breast cancer ranks as one of the most frequently detected forms of cancer in the United States. As per the American Cancer Society (ACS), it is estimated that there were approximately 281,550 new cases of female breast cancer in the country in 2022, making it the most prevalent cancer among American women, second only to skin cancer. Moreover, around 2,650 new cases of breast cancer were diagnosed in men during the same year.

The occurrence of breast cancer varies across different age groups, with the majority of cases being diagnosed in women aged 50 and above. However, it is important to note that younger women and men can also be affected by breast cancer, albeit less frequently.

Although the incidence of breast cancer has remained relatively stable in recent years, there has been a consistent decline in mortality rates. This decline can be attributed to advancements in early detection techniques, a wider range of treatment options, and increased awareness, which has encouraged more women to seek timely medical care.

Breast cancer is a significant global health concern that impacts millions of individuals worldwide. As per the World Health Organization (WHO), breast cancer stands as the most prevalent form of cancer among women on a global scale, regardless of whether they reside in developed or developing nations. In the year 2020, an estimated 2.3 million new cases of female breast cancer were reported globally, representing approximately 11.7% of all newly diagnosed cancer cases.

The occurrence of breast cancer displays regional and population-based disparities, with higher rates documented in North America, Europe, and Australia/New Zealand in comparison to regions such as Africa and Asia. Nevertheless, there has been a gradual rise in the incidence of breast cancer in developing countries, attributed to factors like lifestyle modifications, urbanization, and enhanced detection techniques.

Although breast cancer predominantly affects women, it is crucial to acknowledge that men can also be diagnosed with the disease, albeit less frequently. In 2020, there were an estimated 685,000 new cases of breast cancer identified in men globally.

CHAPTER ONE

Let's Talk About Breast Cancer

An examination of breast cancer covers a range of elements, including epidemiology, risk factors, pathophysiology, clinical presentation, diagnosis, treatment, and prognosis. Here is a summary of each component:

Epidemiology: Breast cancer is the most prevalent cancer in women globally, with millions of new cases identified annually. Incidence rates differ worldwide, with higher rates in developed nations. Nevertheless, incidence is rising in developing regions due to lifestyle changes and enhanced detection methods.

Risk Factors: Several factors can elevate the risk of breast cancer development, such as age, family history, genetic mutations (e.g., BRCA1 and BRCA2), hormonal factors (e.g., early menarche, late menopause), lifestyle factors (e.g., alcohol consumption, obesity), and environmental exposures.

Pathophysiology: Breast cancer originates from abnormal cell growth in breast tissue. It can emerge from ducts (ductal carcinoma) or lobules (lobular carcinoma) and may be influenced by hormonal, genetic, and environmental factors.

Clinical Presentation: Breast cancer can present with various signs and symptoms, including a new lump or mass in the breast or underarm area, changes in breast size or shape, skin changes (e.g., dimpling, redness), nipple changes (e.g., inversion, discharge), and breast pain.

Diagnosis: Diagnosis of breast cancer typically involves a combination of imaging studies (e.g., mammography, ultrasound, MRI) and tissue biopsy to confirm the presence of cancerous cells and determine the cancer's characteristics, such as subtype and stage.

Treatment: Treatment options for breast cancer depend on factors like the cancer's subtype, stage, and individual patient factors. Common treatment methods include surgery (e.g., lumpectomy, mastectomy), chemotherapy, radiation therapy, hormone therapy, targeted therapy (e.g., Herceptin), and immunotherapy.

Prognosis: The prognosis for breast cancer varies based on factors such as the cancer's stage at diagnosis, subtype, and individual patient characteristics.

Discussing breast cancer is essential for multiple reasons:

Awareness: Conversations about breast cancer help to increase awareness regarding the disease, its risk factors, symptoms, and signs. This heightened awareness can empower individuals to identify potential warning signals, seek prompt medical attention, and adopt preventive measures like regular screenings and lifestyle adjustments.

Early Detection: Early detection plays a crucial role in enhancing breast cancer outcomes. By engaging in discussions about breast cancer, we motivate individuals to conduct regular breast self-exams, undergo recommended screening mammograms, and consult healthcare professionals for any worrisome changes in their breast health.

Detecting breast cancer at an early stage significantly boosts the chances of successful treatment and enhances survival rates.

Education: Delving into conversations about breast cancer offers an opportunity to educate the public on various facets of the disease, including risk factors, treatment choices, supportive care services, and survivorship. Education aids in dispelling myths, reducing stigma, and fostering informed decision-making among individuals and communities grappling with breast cancer.

Support: Talking about breast cancer nurtures a supportive atmosphere for individuals grappling with the disease, their loved ones, and caregivers. It promotes open communication, sharing of experiences, and access to resources and support networks that offer emotional, practical, and informational assistance throughout the cancer journey.

Advocacy and Research: Dialogues surrounding breast cancer drive advocacy initiatives aimed at boosting research funding, policy alterations, and enhanced access to quality care for all individuals impacted by the disease. By raising awareness and advocating for increased support and resources, we can advance scientific knowledge, develop innovative treatments, and ultimately strive towards preventing and curing breast cancer.

Breast cancer can manifest differently in each individual, but there are common signs and symptoms to be aware of. These include:

1. Lump or Thickening: The presence of a new lump or mass in the breast or underarm area is often the most noticeable indication of breast cancer. It may feel different from the surrounding tissue or appear thicker than usual.

2. Changes in Breast Size or Shape: Any alterations in the size or shape of the breast, such as swelling, distortion, or asymmetry, should be assessed by a healthcare professional.

3. Changes in Skin Texture: Dimpling, puckering, or ridges on the breast skin that resemble the texture of an orange peel could be an indication of underlying breast cancer.

4. Changes in Skin Color or Appearance: Redness, scaliness, or peeling of the breast skin, particularly around the nipple area, may be signs of breast cancer.

5. Nipple Changes: Changes in the nipple, such as inversion (turning inward), flattening, or discharge (other than breast milk), can be indicative of breast cancer.

6. Breast Pain or Sensitivity: Although breast pain is not typically a common symptom of breast cancer, persistent discomfort or tenderness unrelated to the menstrual cycle should be evaluated.

7. Swelling or Enlargement of One Breast: Unexplained swelling or enlargement of one breast may be a sign of breast cancer, especially if it occurs suddenly or does not resolve over time.

It is crucial to acknowledge that benign conditions can also be responsible for causing these symptoms. However, any changes in the breast should be promptly assessed by a healthcare provider for proper diagnosis and appropriate management. Regular breast self-exams and screening mammograms are also crucial for early detection and improved outcomes in breast cancer.

CHAPTER TWO

Dealing With The Trauma

Breast cancer doesn't mean it's the end of everything. Receiving a diagnosis can be overwhelming, but many individuals lead fulfilling lives after treatment. A breast cancer diagnosis can cause emotional trauma, leading to shock, fear, anxiety, sadness, anger, and uncertainty. Coping with these emotions is crucial for overall well-being. Common responses include shock and denial, fear and anxiety, and sadness and depression. Seeking support from loved ones, healthcare providers, support groups, or mental health professionals can help manage these emotions and promote emotional well-being.

It is completely normal to feel anger or frustration when faced with a breast cancer diagnosis and the potential impact it may have on your life. It is crucial to discover constructive methods for expressing and managing these emotions.This can include talking to a trusted friend or counselor, writing in a journal, or engaging in creative activities such as art or music.

A breast cancer diagnosis can bring about feelings of uncertainty and a loss of control over the future. It is important to focus on what you can control, such as making informed treatment decisions, advocating for your needs, and prioritizing self-care. Practicing mindfulness and acceptance techniques can help cultivate resilience and adaptability in the face of uncertainty.

Seeking support is crucial during this time. Don't hesitate to reach out to loved ones, healthcare providers, support groups, or mental health professionals who can offer understanding, empathy, and practical assistance. Connecting with others who have gone through a similar experience can provide valuable perspective, encouragement, and a sense of solidarity.

Remember that experiencing a range of emotions after a breast cancer diagnosis is completely normal, and seeking support is a sign of strength, not weakness. Taking care of your emotional well-being is an essential part of the healing process as you navigate through treatment, recovery, and survivorship.

The journey towards conquering breast cancer serves as a testament to your unwavering strength, resilience, and determination to triumph over adversity. Although each journey is unique, yours may encompass confronting numerous obstacles, undergoing various treatments, and experiencing a wide range of emotions along the way. Allow me to present a potential account of your remarkable journey:

The commencement of my battle against breast cancer was marked by the shock and disbelief that accompanied the diagnosis. It felt as though my entire world had been upended, leaving me engulfed in fear, uncertainty, and sorrow. Nevertheless, I recognized the necessity of summoning the courage to confront this challenge head-on.

Supported by my loved ones, healthcare professionals, and support networks, I embarked upon a treatment plan tailored to address the specific type and stage of my breast cancer. This plan encompassed surgeries, chemotherapy, radiation therapy, and hormone therapy, with each step presenting its own array of physical and emotional hurdles.

There were moments of uncertainty and desolation, instances when the side effects of treatment seemed insurmountable, and days when I questioned my ability to persevere. However, throughout it all, my determination to fight remained unyielding, as I drew upon the reservoir of inner strength and resilience that resided within me.

CHAPTER THREE

My Journey To Finding A Cure

My journey towards finding a cure for breast cancer was fueled by an unwavering determination to make a meaningful impact in the battle against this destructive illness. Driven by personal encounters, tales of strength, and an unwavering aspiration to establish a future where breast cancer poses no danger, I set out on a mission to propel advancements and breakthroughs in breast cancer research.

Here is a general overview of the typical treatment methods utilized for breast cancer:

Surgical Procedures: Surgery is frequently the primary treatment option for breast cancer and may entail the removal of the tumor and surrounding tissue. The specific type of surgery is determined by various factors, such as the tumor's size and location, the extent of its spread, and the patient's individual preferences. Common surgical interventions for breast cancer include lumpectomy (breast-conserving surgery) and mastectomy (complete breast removal).

Chemotherapy: Chemotherapy involves the use of drugs to eliminate cancer cells or impede their growth and division. It may be recommended prior to or following surgery to reduce tumor size, lower the risk of recurrence, or address cancer that has metastasized to other areas of the body. Chemotherapy regimens vary based on the type and stage of breast cancer and can be administered intravenously or orally.

Radiation Therapy: Radiation therapy employs high-energy beams to target and eradicate cancer cells. It is frequently employed post-surgery (as adjuvant radiation therapy) to eliminate any remaining cancer cells in the breast or nearby lymph nodes and decrease the likelihood of recurrence. Radiation therapy may also be utilized to alleviate symptoms and manage pain in cases of advanced or metastatic breast cancer.

Hormone Therapy: Hormone therapy, also referred to as endocrine therapy, is utilized to treat hormone receptor-positive breast cancer, which constitutes the majority of cases. Hormone therapy functions by obstructing the effects of estrogen or progesterone on cancer cells, thereby slowing tumor growth and reducing the risk of recurrence. Common hormone therapy medications include tamoxifen, aromatase inhibitors, and selective estrogen receptor modulators (SERMs).

Targeted Therapy: Targeted therapy medications are specifically designed to target and attack cancer cells while minimizing harm to healthy cells. They may be used in conjunction with chemotherapy or hormone therapy for specific types of breast cancer, such as HER2-positive breast cancer. Targeted therapy drugs, such as monoclonal antibodies (for example, trastuzumab, pertuzumab), tyrosine kinase inhibitors (like lapatinib), and antibody-drug conjugates (such as ado-trastuzumab emtansine), are part of the treatment arsenal against breast cancer. Immunotherapy, a more recent treatment strategy, utilizes the body's immune system to identify and eliminate cancer cells. Although not yet widely used in breast cancer treatment, immunotherapy drugs like checkpoint inhibitors are under investigation in clinical trials for specific subtypes of breast cancer, notably triple-negative breast cancer (TNBC). Your treatment plan will be tailored to your individual needs, taking into account factors like the stage and subtype of breast cancer, your overall health, personal preferences, and the expertise of your healthcare team. It is crucial to have open discussions with your healthcare providers, actively engage in shared decision-making, and ensure that your treatment plan is in line with your unique needs and priorities.

In addition to the primary treatment modalities mentioned previously, breast cancer treatment may also involve adjunctive or supportive therapies to address symptoms, side effects, and enhance overall well-being. These supportive therapies can complement conventional treatments and improve the quality of life during and after cancer treatment.

1. Pain Management: Breast cancer treatment can lead to pain and discomfort, both during and after the treatment. Pain management techniques may involve medications (like nonsteroidal anti-inflammatory drugs or opioids), nerve blocks, physical therapy, acupuncture, or relaxation methods. It is crucial to communicate any pain or discomfort to your healthcare team for proper management.

2. Nutritional Support: Maintaining proper nutrition is crucial during breast cancer treatment to promote overall health, energy levels, and immune function. A registered dietitian can offer personalized nutrition counseling, suggest dietary changes, and address any nutrition-related side effects of treatment, such as changes in appetite, weight loss, or gastrointestinal problems.

3. Psychosocial Support: Coping with a breast cancer diagnosis and treatment can impact your emotional and mental well-being. Psychosocial support services, like counseling, support groups, and mindfulness-based therapies, can provide emotional support, coping mechanisms, and stress management techniques to navigate the emotional challenges of breast cancer.

4. Fertility Preservation: Certain breast cancer treatments, such as chemotherapy and hormone therapy, may impact fertility in premenopausal women. Fertility preservation options, such as egg or embryo freezing, may be available for women who want to preserve their fertility before starting cancer treatment. It is important to discuss fertility preservation options with your healthcare team before beginning treatment.

5. Physical activity and exercise: These are vital for maintaining strength, mobility, and overall well-being during and after breast cancer treatment. Customized exercise programs that cater to your specific needs and abilities can help manage treatment-related side effects, improve physical function, and enhance emotional well-being.

In addition to traditional treatments, many individuals with breast cancer explore complementary and alternative therapies like acupuncture, massage therapy, yoga, or meditation to alleviate symptoms and improve their quality of life. However, it is crucial to consult with your healthcare team to ensure the safety and effectiveness of these therapies.

6. By incorporating supportive therapies: This can be added into your breast cancer treatment plan, you can address the holistic needs of your body,

mind, and spirit, promoting healing,
resilience, and overall well-being throughout
your journey. Maintaining open
communication with your healthcare team,
actively participating in decision-making,
and adopting a multidisciplinary approach to
care are essential for optimizing outcomes
and enhancing your quality of life during and
after breast cancer treatment.

CHAPTER FOUR

How Can I Prevent It

While it may not always be possible to completely prevent breast cancer, there are measures that individuals can take to decrease their chances of developing the disease. While certain risk factors for breast cancer, such as age, family history, and genetics, cannot be altered, there are lifestyle choices and preventive actions that can help mitigate the risk. Here are some strategies for preventing breast cancer:

1. Maintain a Healthy Lifestyle: Embracing a healthy lifestyle can contribute to reducing the risk of breast cancer. This includes maintaining a healthy weight, engaging in regular physical activity, consuming a well-balanced diet that includes plenty of fruits, vegetables, whole grains, and lean proteins, and limiting alcohol consumption.

2. Limit Hormone Therapy: Prolonged use of hormone replacement therapy (HRT) after menopause has been linked to an increased risk of breast cancer. If considering HRT to manage menopausal symptoms, it is important to discuss the potential risks and benefits with your healthcare provider and explore alternative treatment options.

3. Breastfeed if Possible: Breastfeeding has been shown to lower the risk of breast cancer, particularly if done for an extended period. If you have the opportunity and desire to breastfeed, it is worth considering as it may potentially reduce your risk of developing breast cancer.

4. Stay Physically Active: Engaging in regular physical activity can help decrease the risk of breast cancer. Aim for at least 150 minutes of moderate-intensity exercise or 75 minutes of vigorous-intensity exercise each week, in addition to incorporating strength training exercises at least twice a week.

5. Limit Alcohol Consumption: Consuming alcohol is associated with an increased risk of breast cancer. If you choose to drink alcohol, it is advisable to limit your intake to no more than one drink per day for women and two drinks per day for men.

6.Familiarize Yourself with Your Family's Background: Having knowledge of your family's medical history, particularly regarding breast cancer or genetic mutations like BRCA1 and BRCA2, can heighten the likelihood of developing the disease. If you possess a family history of breast cancer or other risk factors, it is advisable to engage in a conversation with your healthcare provider to assess your risk and explore preventive measures, including genetic counseling and testing.

7.Stay Well-Informed and Advocate for Breast Health: Stay well-informed about the risk factors associated with breast cancer, screening guidelines, and preventive measures. Take an active role in advocating for your breast health by openly discussing any concerns with your healthcare provider, staying updated on recommended screening practices, and advocating for policies and resources that promote breast cancer prevention and early detection efforts.

While these strategies can aid in reducing the risk of breast cancer, it is crucial to remember that they do not guarantee prevention. Regular screening, early detection, and timely treatment continue to be vital components of breast cancer control and management. If you have any concerns regarding your risk of breast cancer or preventive options, seek personalized guidance and recommendations from your healthcare provider.

Let's delve into some additional aspects of breast cancer prevention in greater detail:

Screening and Early Detection: Although screening mammograms cannot prevent breast cancer, they can aid in the early detection of the disease, when it is more treatable. It is important to follow recommended guidelines for breast cancer screening, which include regular mammograms starting at age 40 or earlier for those at higher risk. Additionally, clinical breast exams and breast self-exams are also recommended. Early detection through screening can lead to timely evaluation and treatment, potentially improving outcomes and survival rates.

Chemoprevention: Certain women at an increased risk of breast cancer, such as those with a strong family history or genetic mutations, may be advised to consider chemoprevention medications. These medications, such as selective estrogen receptor modulators (SERMs) or aromatase inhibitors, work by blocking the effects of estrogen on breast tissue, thereby lowering the risk of developing the disease. It is important to discuss the potential benefits and risks of chemoprevention with your healthcare provider to determine if it is the right option for you.

Clinical Trials: Clinical trials play a vital role in advancing breast cancer prevention research by evaluating new preventive strategies, screening methods, and treatment options. Participating in clinical trials not only contributes to scientific knowledge but also provides the opportunity to potentially access novel preventive interventions. Research institutions and cancer centers may offer clinical trials that explore promising new approaches to breast cancer prevention.

Hereditary Risk Assessment: People with strong family history of breast cancer or certain genetic mutations can benefit from genetic counseling and testing. These assessments provide valuable information about inherited risk factors and help guide personalized prevention and screening strategies. A genetic counselor can evaluate your family history, discuss the implications of genetic testing, and offer support and guidance throughout the decision-making process.

Environmental Factors and Lifestyle Changes: While research on the impact of environmental factors on breast cancer risk continues, it is crucial to limit exposure to potential carcinogens and environmental pollutants. Pay attention to household and personal care products that contain chemicals which may disrupt hormonal balance or increase the risk of cancer. Moreover, embracing a healthy lifestyle, such as maintaining a balanced diet, engaging in regular physical activity, managing stress, and avoiding tobacco and excessive alcohol consumption, can aid in lowering the chances of developing breast cancer and enhancing overall well-being.

By integrating these preventive measures into your daily routine and collaborating closely with your healthcare team, you can proactively reduce the likelihood of developing breast cancer and optimize your breast health. Keep in mind that prevention is an ongoing process, and making small adjustments to your habits and behaviors can make a significant difference in decreasing the risk of breast cancer and other chronic illnesses.

CHAPTER FIVE

Conclusion

In summary, breast cancer is a complex disease that impacts millions globally. Despite advancements in understanding, screening, and treatment, it remains a major public health challenge. Early detection, prompt treatment, prevention efforts, and supportive care are crucial for improving outcomes and quality of life for those affected. Continued investment in research, innovation, and advocacy is essential to progress towards a future without breast cancer.

Key Points on Breast Cancer:

Overview of Breast Cancer: Breast cancer is a malignant tumor that forms in the breast tissue, usually originating in the milk ducts or lobules. It is a prevalent cancer in women globally, but it can also impact men.

Factors Influencing Risk: Various factors can elevate the risk of developing breast cancer, such as age, gender, family history, genetic mutations (like BRCA1 and BRCA2), hormonal influences (such as early menstruation, late menopause, and hormone replacement therapy), lifestyle choices (such as obesity, alcohol consumption, and lack of physical activity), and environmental exposures.

Indications and Symptoms: Typical signs and symptoms of breast cancer encompass a lump or mass in the breast or underarm region, alterations in breast size or shape, nipple discharge (not related to breastfeeding), breast pain or discomfort, skin changes (like redness, dimpling, or thickening), and swelling or inflammation of the breast tissue.

Detection and Screening: The diagnosis of breast cancer usually involves a blend of imaging tests (such as mammography, ultrasound, and MRI), biopsy (for analyzing tissue samples), and laboratory assessments (to evaluate hormone receptor status and genetic mutations). Regular breast cancer screening, including mammograms and clinical breast exams, is crucial for early identification and management.

Therapeutic Approaches: The treatment of breast cancer is contingent on various factors, including cancer type and stage, tumor characteristics, and individual patient considerations. Common treatment options consist of surgery (like lumpectomy or mastectomy), chemotherapy, radiation therapy, hormone therapy, targeted therapy, and immunotherapy. Treatment strategies are tailored to meet the specific needs and preferences of each patient.

Prevention: Although it may not always be possible to completely prevent breast cancer, there are measures individuals can take to lower their chances of developing the disease. These include maintaining a healthy lifestyle by managing weight, staying physically active, eating a balanced diet, limiting alcohol intake, and avoiding tobacco. It is also important to be aware of your family history and genetic risk factors, undergo regular breast cancer screening, and consider preventive measures like chemoprevention and genetic counseling/testing.

Support and Awareness: Breast cancer diagnosis and treatment can have significant physical, emotional, and psychosocial impacts on individuals and their families. Seeking support from healthcare providers, support groups, and mental health professionals is crucial. Additionally, raising awareness about breast cancer risk factors, screening guidelines, and prevention strategies is important.

By staying well-informed, taking proactive steps to reduce risk, undergoing regular screening, and seeking support when needed, individuals can empower themselves to effectively manage breast cancer and promote overall breast health. Early detection and treatment play a vital role in improving outcomes and survival rates for those diagnosed with breast cancer.

www.ingramcontent.com/pod-product-compliance
Lightning Source LLC
Chambersburg PA
CBHW070752260726
48660CB00007B/3086